Weight Loss

All the Truth about Popular Diets You Wish You Knew

Table Of Contents

Introduction

Congratulations on downloading this book and thank you for doing so. The best description of diet is a fixed plan of drinking and eating where the amount and type of food are planned out in order to achieve some target like weight loss or maintaining optimal health. It is a well-known fact that typical western meals are too high in sweet, salt, and fried foods. In the long term, such a way of eating raises person risks of obesity, numerous diseases and dying early.

Some of the weight loss diet plans promise to help you lose weight very fast. If you are overweight, aim to lose about 10% of the starting weight by losing ½ - 1 kilo a week. You did not gain 10 kilos overnight; it took time. The same thing goes for losing 10 kilos. Otherwise, you eventually end up putting the weight back on.

Most of us need to eat less and get more physically active. We gain weight when the amount of energy we consume exceeds the amount of energy we burn through exercise and usual everyday activities. Indeed, calories matter, but focusing on nutritional content is an important part of promoting weight loss too.

So called, "macronutrient management"-style diets have become mainstream when talking about optimal eating plans. Researchers have begun comparing low-fat to low-carbohydrate diets in order to determine which is most efficient. Results of studies show that while a particular diet plan may lead to weight loss for one person, it may just not be effective for another person. There is no one perfect diet for everyone due to individual differences in lifestyle and genes.

Atkins Diet

In the 70s Dr. Robert Atkins developed the weight loss program which for now is one of the most widely recognized low-carb diets. This diet plan includes four phases. During the induction phase, you are keeping net carbs at the lowest level for two weeks or longer; it is about only 25g daily. Phase one is designed for rapid weight loss and during second (balancing) phase more carbs are slowly added with the aim to find the best carbohydrate balance. On third or fine tuning stage you can make small tweaks to reach a healthy weight for life. And the name of the fourth phase is lifetime maintenance; you should continue eating a healthy diet with limited carbohydrates to maintain your goal weight. If you prefer a structured eating plan, the Atkins diet will work for you. Here are some additional reasons that Atkins might work for you:

Some people have lost a lot of weight on the Atkins diet plan. During the first stage of the diet, rapid weight loss is a common thing. This early weight loss can be motivating and provide a boost of confidence.

Some people like the fact that you can eat more red meat, cheese, butter, and cream on the Atkins diet. Apparently, it is one of the diets that appeals most to males.

On this plan, you can define your ideal carb-intake level. You don't have to count calories; you should worry about carbohydrates only.

You are likely to cut your sugar intake which may lead to improvements in your health. Also, the Atkins diet eliminates most processed carbs and alcohol. Instead, you will be encouraged to consume healthy carbohydrates, especially in the later phases of the diet plan.

Atkins diet cons.

The high intake of red meat, processed meat, and saturated fat may increase your risk of heart disease. Also, there are some concerns about the advice to add salt, which is in contradiction with current health information.

Some people experienced severe discomfort as a result of the dietary changes in the eating plan. Just because our typical menu is full of carbohydrates, it can be challenging to make decrease intake of carbs significantly from the start. Probably, you should choose a diet plan that starts with small changes.

Initial side effects can include fatigue, poor mood, headache, bad breath, nausea, insomnia, dizziness and constipation from cutting out carbohydrates, and potentially for lower fiber intake. In order to avoid dehydration, you should drink plenty of water during the first phase of the Atkins program. Choose your carbs carefully; you still need a fiber which promotes bowel movements and healthy digestion. While the Atkins plan allows you to drink tea or black coffee, you should watch your caffeine intake. If you consume too much caffeine, you may become dehydrated and get constipated as a result.

Dieters who return to eating carbohydrates without restriction usually gain back all of the weight they lost during the diet, and sometimes even more. In some cases, too strict diet plan leads to food binges, feeling guilty and weight gain.

Keto Diet

Initially, keto diet was used as a treatment for childhood epilepsy. Ketosis is a state in which human body burns fats for fuel, instead of carbohydrates. This phenomenon is possible when your carb intake is very low. Most of the children who follow keto diet experience significant improvement of their state. And more than 10% may even stop suffering epileptic seizures completely. During ketosis our liver releases in the blood specific molecules – ketones. Supposedly, ketones may cause a change in brain chemistry that limits epileptic fits. Obviously, you should consult a doctor before attempting the ketogenic diet.

The ketogenic diet is extremely low in carbohydrates; it's about 5% of total daily calorie intake. That means that you are allowed to eat a minimal amount of low-carb vegetables, such as leafy greens, broccoli, cabbage, cucumber, celery, tomatoes, peppers, asparagus, and zucchini. Furthermore, keto diet includes less protein than others low carb diets – usually about 20%. So, you can eat a moderate amount of protein, such as eggs, poultry, meat, and seafood. Remaining 75% of your calories are represented by fats; this diet is really high fat. In other words, you should consume a significant amount of high-fat food, such as cheese, butter, bacon, egg yolks, nuts, coconut milk, avocado, olive oil, and any other oil.

On a ketogenic diet, you are not allowed to eat most processed foods, fruits, grains, starchy vegetables, slightly-sweet vegetables, grains, beans, and legumes.

So, what about benefits of a ketogenic diet for losing weight? Undoubtedly, this kind of diet improves our body's ability to exploit stored fat as an energy resource. Indeed, your ability to convert fat into fuel substantially decreases if you eat a high-carb meal. However, our body simply has no other option than turning to fats for energy in the state of ketosis.

Supposedly, your appetite decreases in the state of ketosis. Some experts claim that you are able to survive on fewer calories and won't feel hungry. It is an interesting fact that ketosis happens when levels of blood ketones are higher than normal either during fasting or starvation or when your carbohydrates intake is very low. That means that some health benefits of fasting may be due to ketosis itself. And ketogenic diet is an attempt to get the health effects of fasting without actually fasting.

Ketogenic diet cons

Consuming a high-fat diet can be detrimental to our long-term health. Probably, the alteration in your blood lipid profile is a major concern in keto diet. Statistical data indicate that altered blood lipid profile raises cholesterol levels in some people whereas it lowers in others. Foods like egg yolks, lard, bacon, and butter are high in saturated fat, which can increase your risk of heart disease.

Strict limiting plant foods can result in deficiencies of some micronutrients. In order to prevent this, you should consider taking high-quality vitamin and mineral supplements on a daily basis. Also, you will need dietary fiber supplements for your digestive system proper functioning.

As you can see, keto diet has highly restrictive nutritional guidelines, and it can be challenging to adhere to a diet plan that induces ketosis. Moreover, if you like to eat out, you should know that it's difficult to find appropriate foods at restaurants, school, and other social functions. If you use keto diet for weight loss and don't need to be in ketosis for epilepsy management, you may be more tempted to give up.

Extreme lowering carb intake seems to have more adverse effects for women. Many women have found that ketogenic diet that worked perfectly for their husband didn't work for them. For some woman, being in ketosis creates an issue with the hypothalamus, which is partly responsible for the hormones responsible for the menstrual cycle. As well, following low carbohydrate diet plan can disrupt the leptin and thyroid. Your carbs may be just too low for you.

South Beach Diet

The South Beach Diet was originally developed for heart patients to help them lower their risk of developing cardiovascular disease. This diet plan was created by cardiologist Dr. Arthur Agatston and dietician Marie Almon, and the scheme looks pretty similar to the Atkins program at some points. Both the Atkins and South Beach diets focus on a low-carb nutritional plan, which the authors of each diet claim will help you lose excess weight. Also, just like Atkins program, the South Beach diet unfolds in three distinct stages.

Phase one is intended to eliminate cravings and stabilize blood sugar. It lasts two weeks, and it is the shortest and most restrictive phase. You cannot eat sugary foods, starches, grains, fruits, pasta, and bread. Alcohol is banned too. So you will eat generous portions of lean protein with some low-GI veggies and low-fat dairy. If you have less than 10 lb to lose, you can start from the second phase, which is less restrictive.

In phase two "good carbohydrates" are reintroduced into your menu. In addition to the menu of the first phase, you can eat now most fruits, starches and whole-grain bread and pasta. This step lasts until you reach your target weight.

Phase three is the maintenance stage and is your lifelong way to eat. So you should continue to make proper food choices for the rest of the life. No major food groups are off-limits, and low-GI carbs, vegetables, and fruits are recommended.

After phase one, the South Beach Diet provides a balanced diet and doesn't require any strict portion sizes, counting calories, fat grams, carbohydrates or anything else. Still,

South Beach is lower in carbs and higher in protein and healthy fats than the usual American diet.

The South Beach Diet is meant to be easy to follow. You are encouraged to eat three meals and healthy mid-morning and mid-afternoon snacks a day so that you won't get hungry.

Also, you will learn to choose the right carbs and the right fats; it can be a kind of crash course on nutrition. According to the South Beach Diet, carbohydrates with a high glycemic index are bad. Bad carbohydrates break down too quickly and flood your blood with excessive sugar. In order to regulate the blood sugar, your body releases high amounts of hormone insulin into the blood. Insulin stops burning body's fat and instead, activates accumulating the unused sugar as fat. The more high-GI carbs you eat, the more you crave them. Foods which contain that type of carbohydrates are usually sweets, processed foods, such as refined sugars and processed grains. On the other hand, fruits and vegetables are good sources of carbs because they are high in fiber, as well as vitamins and minerals. Low-GI carbohydrates provide a more constant flow of glucose into the bloodstream; that keeps you energized for longer. In addition, eating good carbs reduces hunger, helps you eat less, declines risk of diabetes, and improve a level of blood cholesterol.

Also, the South Beach replaces foods heavy in saturated and trans-fats (bad) with food rich in omega-3 fatty acids and unsaturated fats (good).

The primary advantage to following the program is its emphasis on building healthy habits that will help you achieve a target weight and maintain it. We know that physical exercise should be an essential component of any weight loss program. Fitness aspect of this program is represented in two forms. The first form is an interval walking, which means alternating between slow and very fast pace. The second form is a full body workout with an accent on your core. You should work out every day for 20 mins, shifting between these two ways. And "The South Beach Diet Supercharged" plan offers some tips on customizing the program to your fitness level.

Optional online membership in South Beach Diet costs 5 dollars a week and the first week is free. Online members can use the company's website to track their diet and weight goals, meals, and shopping-list generator. Also, South Beach dieters communicate with each other via discussion boards, and a daily newsletter provides them with the new recipes. Moreover, the company has a line of high-protein and meal bars, snack-sized smoothies. All products are free of artificial flavors and sweeteners.

South Beach Diet cons

In terms of health concerns, the first phase appears to be most problematic. As we have already heard, strict limiting of your carbohydrate intake can cause developing ketosis. And ketosis can cause dehydration, gastrointestinal problems, weakness, dizziness, and fatigue. Eliminating fruits, whole grains and cereals during this phase will result in loss of fiber, vitamins, and minerals.

There is no sufficient scientific data on the South Beach diet. We have only one study that Dr. Agatston conducted with his own patients. The patient-sample was not very large, and it was not a long-term study.

This program uses the glycemic index as a basis for making food choices, which can be inaccurate sometimes. For instance, the GI is variable with the way of preparing food, ripeness, and many other factors. Popular insulin hypothesis is dramatically oversimplified. Insulin is not only storage hormone; it's rather an anabolic hormone. That means that we need insulin along with testosterone and growth hormone to create a muscle-building, anabolic environment.

The China Study

The China-Cornell-Oxford Project was one of the largest extensive studies of the relationship between human nutrition and chronic diseases such as cancer, diabetes, and coronary heart disease. The China Study was launched via the Chinese Academy of Preventive Medicine, Cornell University, and Oxford University. Scientific data collected over a span of 20 years result in "more than 8000 statistically significant associations between lifestyle, diet, and disease variables." The study included 367 variables and 6500 adults from 65 counties in China.

One of the project's directors T. Colin Campbell, Ph.D., and his son, Thomas M. Campbell II, MD, analyze and discuss the data from this study and other nutritional research and recommend their version for the best diet plan for long-term health. The scientists conclude that people who eat plant-based, whole-food, vegan diet will escape or reverse the development of numerous illnesses. In "The China Study" book they write that "eating foods that contain any cholesterol above 0 mg is unhealthy." Also, authors say that diets like Atkins or South Beach can have dangerous consequences for long-term health.

Vegan Diet

Vegan diet strictly relies on plant-based, whole, foods such as vegetables, fruits, nuts, seeds, legumes, whole grains, and beans. Vegans abstain from eating any animal products such as meats, poultry, fish, seafood, eggs, dairy, honey, and any prepared foods containing these ingredients. Moreover, vegans also avoid animal products in other domains. For instance, they do not wear leather and fur or use makeup that has used animal ingredients in the manufacturing process.

Concern for the environment and compassion for animals are two core vegan values. Evidence suggests that factory farming and industrial fishing has negative ecological impacts. The current vegan movement has brought attention to the inappropriate treatment of farm animals. Some of them are so unwell that they can't even stand on their own feet. This is not only unethical, but factory farming produces foods that come from sick animals and are high in inflammatory compounds that are associated with increased risk of cancer and heart disease.

Apparently, vegans are significantly thinner than other vegetarians and much thinner much thinner than those who eat meat. And the lower body weight is associated with a lower risk of diabetes and cancer. Other health benefits of the vegan diet include lower cholesterol, better blood pressure, and cardiovascular health. These health advantages can be explained by the fact that vegan diet is low in saturated fat and cholesterol-free. On the other hand, consuming larger volumes of whole plant-based foods, vegans receive greater amounts of dietary fiber, health-promoting phytochemicals, potassium and magnesium, folic acid and the antioxidant vitamins C and E. And antioxidants are vital because they protect our cells from free radicals caused by many factors.

Vegan diet cons

While nutrition experts agree about good vegan resources for most necessary nutrients, the proper planning is the key factor here. Most vegans struggle with consuming adequate amounts of protein. Your diet should incorporate some protein into every meal. Since vegans avoid typical protein sources like eggs and meat, they have to incorporate it through other means. Best plant-based protein sources include nuts, beans, seeds, legumes, and some whole grains such as quinoa.

Avoid overly-processed meat substitutes, which can be packed with preservatives and sodium. Many seemingly vegan foods contain ingredients like whey or gelatin. Whey is derived from milk and gelatin is derived from meat, so they are not suitable for a vegan diet. And beware refined carbohydrates and other highly processed foods. You shouldn't consume junk-food just because it is labeled "vegan."

Vegan diet poses a risk for micronutrient deficiencies. In particular, vegans need to be conscious of omega-3 fatty acids, vitamins B12 and D, calcium, iodine, iron, and zinc. According to the Academy of Nutrition and Dietetics, all these nutrients can be sourced without the use of animal products. However, in some cases supplementation may be necessary. For example, vitamin B12 occurs naturally in animal foods only; vegans should use nutritional yeasts and fortified products.

Also, it may be challenging to choose from the menu when dining out.

Other Vegetarian Diets

Term "vegetarian" broadly refers to individuals who restrict consumption of animal foods and primarily rely on whole plant-based products for a living. Vegan is the most restrictive version of plant-based diets. There are at least three other kinds of vegetarian diet: Lacto-vegetarian, Ovo-vegetarian, and lacto-ovo-vegetarian.

Lacto-vegetarians don't consume meat, fish, poultry or eggs. However, they readily consume milk and dairy products like cheese and yogurt. Most of the vegetarians in South Asia are Lacto-vegetarians.

Ovo-vegetarians do not consume meat, fish, poultry, and dairy; but they allow themselves to consume eggs.

Lacto-ovo-vegetarians consume dairy and eggs but exclude meat, fish, and poultry. This type of vegetarian is most common across the globe.

Individuals who follow vegetarian eating patterns are less likely to become obese than people who don't follow such patterns. Partly, this may be the result of higher consumption of low-calorie and more filling foods such as veggies, fruits, beans and whole grains. On the flip side, cutting out high-calorie foods such as fatty meats and lard can result in a lower in calories intake. In addition, some health experts suggest that using of spices such as onions, garlic, ginger, and turmeric to flavor foods protects the consumer against stroke, heart disease, and cancer.

Lacto-ovo-vegetarian diet can be sufficient in vitamin B12 and most other essential nutrients. Adequate protein consumption is not a problem too.

Despite the numerous potential health benefits of vegetarian diet, these positive effects are not automatic. They are more likely to occur when you stick with mainly whole, fresh and healthy foods. Some people gain weight on a vegetarian diet because all they eat is rice, bread, and pasta. A vegetarian diet that relies on sweets, solid fats, sugar-sweetened beverages and refined grains can be unhealthier than a diet that includes meat. Technically speaking, doughnuts, candy bars, and French fries are vegetarian. However, these foods can contain dangerous trans fats, which lower your levels of "good" cholesterol and raise your unhealthy LDL cholesterol. It's not what we expect from the vegetarian diet, right?

Battle of the Macronutrients

The low-carb and low-fat diet movements have focused on what macronutrient we should rely on as our main energy source. The problem with that is that we all have different genes from each other, and different lifestyles, with different activity levels, and metabolism. Moreover, you may have different needs at different times of your life. That's awesome if you found a particular nutritional idea – like vegetarianism or Atkins – helped you achieve your goals. However, it doesn't mean everyone else should follow the same diet plan; it works personally for you, under a certain set of circumstances, at one point in your life. There is no a single best diet for absolutely every person to follow, forever and always.

In reality, the human body is incredibly adaptable and can do well under a host of different dietary conditions. For instance, the African Masai and Arctic Inuit eat a lot of animal products and fat with very few vegetables. At the same time, Kitavans in the South Pacific eat mostly vegetables and starchy carbohydrates; their fat consumption is low. All these traditional diets of various ethnic groups and tribes throughout the world provide people with relatively good health; incidences of obesity, diabetes, cardiovascular disease are minimal. So, the human race can eat just about any diet and keep growing and reproducing.

How can so much different nutritional approaches all promote good health and longevity? You probably will be surprised, but most effective diet plans are more similar than different. Even low-carb and plant-based eating programs are not as different as we might think. Both dietary philosophies raise nutritional awareness, improve food quality, and help control appetite.

Simply caring more about what you are eating is a key factor in whether you will get lean, lose weight, and improve your health. On the low-carbohydrates diet, you have to eat more natural, free-range animal-based foods that are minimally processed. According to the vegan diet plan, you have to eat more natural plant based foods that are higher in antioxidants, fiber and are minimally processed. As we can see, each camp recommends consuming nutrient-rich, whole and minimally processed foods. And this is the crucial nutritional intervention which is more important than fat, carb, and protein breakdowns. Apparently, shifting away from highly processed foods eliminates deficiencies of some nutrients such as water, proteins, certain vitamins and minerals, and essential fatty acids. When we are deficient in essential nutrients, we feel, look, and perform just awfully.

When we are more aware of what we are eating, choose higher quality foods, and eliminate deficiencies, we most likely end up eating less total food. Usually, focusing on food quality and food awareness is enough for you to tune into your own appetite and hunger.

Demonizing some foods or macronutrients gets attention, sells books, and gives good TV. However, humans have adapted to do well under almost all sorts of dietary conditions. While some of us are going to feel great eating mostly starch and some just as great eating mostly meat and fat, the simple truth for most of us is in the middle.

IIFYM: If It Fit Your Macros

IIFYM recommends getting 50% of your calories from healthy carbohydrates, 30% of calories from protein, and the rest from healthy fats. Basically, if your food falls within that breakdown and you stay within your daily caloric budget, you will lose weight or stay fit. It works just because it follows a fundamental weight-loss rule: eat fewer calories than your body needs.

This popular diet strategy allows you the flexibility to eat your favorite foods while still losing weight. And we know that having some flexibility in your diet is a key factor for the long-term success. That is not a free pass to eat nothing but cake and hamburgers. It just means that you can work treats into your diet plan, by taking a special approach to food and nutrition. Obviously, you can't have half of your food as cake and expect to look good and feel good.

The major benefit of the IIFYM diet approach is that it doesn't have to interfere with our social and dating life. It's not much fun explaining that you only eat healthy food on your first date. Not having to worry about your clean diet in a dating world is a lot easier.

 On the other hand, you should remember about hormonal consequences to eating a particular food at an appropriate time. For instance, consuming a bunch of sugar before you go to bed is going to switch off the production of human growth hormone and spike your insulin. HGH is one of the most fat-burning hormones in your body, so we are interested in maximizing its production and presence.

Although IIFYM allows you enjoy whatever food you want as long as you stay within calorie and macros limits, sometimes it is not easy to track macronutrients and calories. Obviously, you should limit your portions sizes of junk foods in order to follow this diet plan successfully. However, controlling portions is a big problem for many people. Overweight people tend to eat larger portions and larger meals. As a result, they often make mistakes counting their energy intake.

As an IIFYM fan, you can choose less healthy options like refined carbohydrates instead of whole grains and fruit juices instead of whole fruits. Undoubtedly, eating a lot of these foods will impact your weight-loss progress, your health, and your energy levels.

Weight Watchers

Weight Watchers positions their self as providing a lifestyle program, not just another variety of diet. That's why I'm going to provide a more detailed analysis here. You see, it's a much trickier thing; it is a business of behavior change. You should realize that your target is not hitting the certain weight, but rather building new eating and fitness habits. This kind of approach will allow you to benefit for a lifetime.

Weight Watchers diet is well researched and classified as top grade compared to most others. For instance, British Medical Research Council provided two studies; results of which tell us that Weight Watchers regimen is an effective way to lose weight. These studies were not a single attempt to investigate so much popular weight loss plan. Indeed, if you look through the list of best weight loss diets, you will find Weight Watchers program amid the top-ranked ones.

One of the serious medical periodicals 'Annals of Internal Medicine' published the curious report on this subject. According to it, eleven general weight loss plans have been studied with a randomized controlled trial. Weight Watchers program was one of two diets which indicated that participants lost more weight over one year than people sticking to their own diet. It is evidence beyond a reasonable doubt, isn't it? So, how is it possible to outperform other popular commercial weight loss strategies?

Four pillars of the Weight Watchers program are behavior, food, exercise, and support. WW focuses on modifying diet and encouraging physical activity to create an energy deficit. Experts say that your diet is 80% responsible for obtaining a desirable result in weight loss. So, this program works blending nutrition points-driven plan with a strong group support system and inspiration to exercise. The program offers you an education on cooking, nutrition, and lifestyle.

Also, the WW program teaches you portion control. In order to count your Smart points accurately, you need to learn how to measure your food portions correctly. This skill is important, and it will be significant for whole your life.

Weight Watchers have their own line of foods that you can buy in the supermarkets. However, you are not required to purchase these products to join the Weight Watchers program. Also, the company provides a broad range of services including digital systems and apps to monitor weight change, energy intake and outlet, as well recipes and healthy meal ideas. For instance, if you are preparing a meal that is not listed in the Weight Watchers database, you can calculate the Smart-points value by ingredients with the help of appropriate mobile app or through the Weight Watchers website.

I have to recognize I am not a huge fan of calories counting. In fact, it's annoying and stressful task; a kind of heavy duty as for me. Also, it's not very easy to count calories accurately. We all are looking for perfect accuracy, aren't we? So, finding only close match leads to some frustration. As a result, we tend to give up on calorie counting and on attempts to lose weight altogether.

Besides, you should think long term about the weight loss process. Are you ready to count calories every day of your life? If you are not, then do not even bother starting. Anyone can restrict his calorie intake thanks to a temporary diet, but when you stop, you will gain it again. Actually, your success here is measured by not only the amount of weight you have lost but rather on how long you keep it off.

It is well known that Weight Watchers program uses the own point-based system. Every food is given a certain point value based on nutritional value. That means it is no longer necessary to count calories like most of other diets require you to do. Instead of this, you have to keep track of points.

The information about the Smart-points value of different food products is available through Weight Watchers apps and online. Naturally, the exact formula for Smart-points calculating is not available. However, you can find a few variants of a rough formula made by mathematic enthusiasts. I have found that this one looks most close to the original Smart-point formula:

$$SP = (Calories + Sugar*4 + Saturated\ Fat*9 - Protein*3.2)/33$$

Supposedly this formula could be applied to any food or recipe with nutrition facts information. But fruit and vegetable exception makes it impossible in many cases to calculate Smart-points scrupulously. For instance, restaurant disclosure data includes veggies in the numbers.

Depending on your weight, your goal, age, gender, and your level of activity you are allowed a particular number of points per day. Obviously, knowing your Smart Point daily budget is very important.

Criteria (Step One)	Points	Example
Female	2	
Male	8	2
Nursing Female (additional 12 on top of the 2)	12	
Age (Step Two)		
17 - 26	4	
27 - 37	3	
38 - 47	2	2
48 - 57	1	
58 and over	0	
Weight – (Step Three) Take the first two numbers of your weight and add them to the points you already have from Steps one and two. Here are some examples.		
150 – 159 pounds	15	
170 – 179 pounds	17	17
190 - 199 pounds	19	
200 – 209 pounds	20	
230 – 239 pounds	23	
300 – 309 pounds and so on	30	
Height – (Step Four)		
Under 5 feet	0	
5.0 – 5.9 feet	1	1
5.10 and over	2	
Daily Activity Level (Step Five)		
Most of the day sitting (desk job)	0	0
Most of the day on your feet	2	
Most of the day walking	4	
Work hard physically throughout the day	6	
Final Daily Points Score		22
Presto! You have now calculated your points and are on your way.		

Also, it is interesting to know how Points system evolves over time. Initially, Weight Watchers point system stimulated to cut fats and consume fiber. Point Plus system added protein in the equation. In December 2015, Smart Points replaced Point Plus. The new scheme still guides users toward an eating pattern that is higher in protein. The distinctive feature of Smart Point system is stringent penalizing for high-sugar and high-saturated fat consumption. Obviously, now calories content is not the one and only criteria to base your food choices on. For instance, fiber in your meal will keep you feeling full longer, which can prevent you from ingesting more calories. But fiber is absent in the Smart Point formula. That's why most fresh fruits and vegetables are zero points in the Smart Points system.

On the other hand, point restrictions for eating pastries and cookies are pretty high on the new program. Of cause, there were some people who had worries that Smart Points system lacks flexibility in a food-point assignment. However, can you disagree with the fact that an apple and banana are much healthier and more nutrient-packed choices than cake and candy bar?

Exercising is the next vital factor to success in loses weight process. Every type of physical activity is also given a Fit Points value; in this way, you are rewarded for exercising. If you don't know where to start, Weight Watchers program will help you to uncover many different ways to earn activity points. Things like walking the dog, dancing, housecleaning, playing golf, bowling, gardening and yard work will get you some extra points. And certainly, you shouldn't forget to count your aerobics and weight lifting training.

Also, you can swap Fit Points for food if needed. Regular physical activity helps prevent many health issues, improves sleep quality, and makes you feel better. After your training session, you may find yourself more optimistic and less stressed. That's because good workout stimulates the release of endorphins and others feel-good brain chemicals. Besides that, regular exercising can increase your confidence. So, if swapping works well for you, you can do it since these points are what you earn for being active. However, if you cannot reach the result you want, you should refuse from swapping.

Fit points calculation formula takes into account your weight, the duration, and intensity of your physical activity. Actually, the formula is pretty simple for understanding:

Fit Points = weight in lbs*duration in minutes*intensity factor

The intensity factor of a particular form of physical activity varies between individuals. It depends on a people exercise experience and their current level of fitness.

In order to define the intensity factor of your workout just keep an eye on your breathing patterns and sweating. So, a low-intensity workout does not change your breathing pattern, and you are not sweating doing it. If you are not used to physical exercising, low-intensity training sessions are a right place to start. Yoga practice or simply stretching routine, as well as light walking, could be good examples of low-intensity exercise. Of course, each of these exercises might provide either low or moderate intensity training, depending on the pace that you use.

A moderate intensity workout makes your breathing deep and often, but you are not out of breath. It feels somewhat hard and results in a light sweating after about ten mins of training.

A high-intensity workout seems challenging; you develop a sweat after 3 to 5 minutes. The 'talk test' shows that you can't say more than a few words at a time without pausing for breath. Examples of high-intensity exercise include fast swimming, strength workout with free weights and weight machines, or activities that use a weight of you own body – such as calisthenics, rock climbing, or heavy gardening.

You need to choose the type of training that suits your level of fitness. If you are not sure what your intensity factor should be, talk to your physician. If you are new to workout, start at a light intensity and gradually build up to a moderate intensity session.

The more intense and longer your physical activity, the more fat you burn. However, balance is still necessary. Overdoing of physical training will increase the risk of injury and overtraining. So, don't push yourself too fast, too hard; just be realistic. Fitness is a lifetime marathon, not a sprint to a finish line. The basic rule here is "don't give up." You can change exercise, workout plan and intensity factor depending on the goal and mood, but physical activity must always be present in your life.

The benefits of 'going beyond the comfort zone' could be interesting for advanced fitness practitioners in order to increase their performance level. The point is not only to go somewhere but also to stay there, making discomfort zone your new comfort level. Human is a highly adaptive beast; we could adapt to some level of the discomfort too!

When you reach your weight loss goal, you should figure out your new Smart-points budget. Apparently, you need more points to stop losing weight. Also, you enter a so-called maintenance period which lasts six weeks. Now your goal is maintaining weight instead of losing, and you have to be focused on this aim. During this time there will be regular weight-ins. If you stay within two pounds of your goal weight in that six week period, you will be promoted to a Lifetime Member. Lifetime members can participate in any meeting free. However, they must stay within two pounds of their weight, so they have to weigh-in at least once a month.

In reality, available statistic shows us that average weight losses achieved through Weight Watchers program are modest relative to common anticipations. According to one of the studies mentioned above, in one year's time, on Weight Watchers, participants lost an average of twelve pounds only. But that's just average numbers.

The bottom line is that program works well for people who are health conscious. And unfortunately, the program is not going to work fine in a long-term perspective for partakers who are less health conscious. Health conscious individuals are concerned with nutrition, stress, physical activity, and their environment. Also, they accept responsibility for their health and living with healthy habits. In order to become more health conscious, you should learn what healthy and unhealthy practices are.

Your environment defines your success. Does it sound familiar? That means that in order to be successful you need to spend some of your time in a company of people who support and encourage your efforts toward your goal.

Indeed, support is a significant component of Weight Watchers program. Humans are social animals, and weekly group meeting made us feel more accountable for our weight loss efforts. Clearly, people in a group-based program are much more engaged and have a better success rate. Supposedly, group support is also effective for long-term behavioral changes and steady weight loss results.

Usually, schedule of the meeting includes weigh-ins, group discussion about both scale and non-scale problem solving, and sharing best practices. Group membership may vary from week to week, but the leader of the group is a permanent person who has successfully completed Weight Watchers program and received training from the company. Only your group leader and you see what the scales say, so please don't worry about the public humiliating weigh-in.

Also, all Weight Watchers members have access to an online 24/7 Expert Chat. Another innovation in the area of community and support is a phone-based coaching program. You have great opportunity to choose your own personal coach, work through your worksheet and create your own personalized action plan.

The Weight Watchers program is for women; it just doesn't appeal to males. It seems like about 90% of participants at Weight Watchers meetings are female. Weight loss is a regular topic for women to discuss; it's their shared purpose. I suppose meeting and talking about weight loss are just natural things for any women.

Any man with overweight could face health issues like impotence, heart disease, diabetes, and cancer. Apparently, men also could benefit from Weight Watchers program. Even more, the company provides weight loss plan, customized for guys. And online consulting is an available substitution for live meetings.

The Weight Watchers program is not free. So many people like almost everything about WW except the cost. Indeed, after not losing weight for a couple of weeks, paying for the program can feel completely stupid.

One the other hand, you have no contract with Weight Watchers; it's just a "pay-as-you-go" membership. Yeah, you have to pay, but this is for your health. So, spending money on WW program is not a waste; it's a smart investment.

Sometimes you choose foods that are not very healthy and nutritious. Well, this is the other side of "no food is off limits" WW principle. For instance, it could seem like a waste to use your Smart points for healthy olive oil, when you could spend them on not-so-healthy cheese or bread.

Everything in Moderation, Including Fad Diets

Apparently, meal plan has long been a usual tool of the nutrition and weight-loss industry. So, experts are taught to create meal plans, and dieters expect them and accept them with enthusiasm. However, a meal plan can be really hard to follow, no matter how motivated you are. Our life just corrects our eating plan under many circumstances, such as special holiday or someone's birthday, we are expected to work late, and we are not always prepared, offsprings get sick, and so on.

A meal plan is meant to be a short-term tool. Most meal plans are designed to help you get a particular short-term goal, like dropping a few extra pounds before a photo session or cutting weight for a sports competition. But if you are too strict for too long, you're not likely to keep living that way. Often we eat meals with other people. Also, we eat meals that match our social interests and cultural background. Food is not only a fuel source; it serves us in festivity, it's the oldest social network in our world. Indeed, if your diet plan takes those roles of food away from you, the likelihood of you sticking with it is really low.

Some authors of recent diet studies come to the similar conclusion about popular diet plans: choose any program that you will stick to. Evaluate your individual preferences and your lifestyle to find a diet that you can maintain for a long enough period.

Unfortunately, weight regain is a serious problem that many dieters underestimate. According to the one University of California, even after losing weight, 30-65% of dieters gain back more weight than they actually had lost. Obviously, weight regain is just a result of giving up on your diet after "hitting-finish-line." That's why it's so important to find a way of eating which becomes your new normal way of life and happens to improve weight loss.

For the majority of people, diets don't lead to sustained results in weight loss or health benefits. Any diet study of less than 2 years is too short to show whether participants have gained back the weight they lost. And evidence shows us that repeatedly gaining and losing weight is linked to heart diseases, diabetes, stroke, and altered immune function.

Small Changes, Healthy Habits, and Lifestyle

Fad diets don't help you stay slim in the long term. So what does work? Long-term eating habits always trump popular diets and meal plans. The best approach is not a diet only but a way of life that includes healthy food you enjoy, exercise, and healthy habits. It addresses not just losing weight, but also health.

Usually, when you start paying attention to your eating, you start thinking about physical exercise too. In fact, many of diet programs recommend regular physical activity. Working out dramatically improves your body's ability to turn the food you eat into functional muscle tissue instead of extra fat.

Your diet plan should involve making many small changes in different areas, rather than a single extreme change in one area. Just think how you could make a little bit healthier the menu you are already eating. Make small improvements to what you normally eat and enjoy, one step at a time. For example, eating vegetables and fruits at every meal, not letting yourself get too hungry between meals, and limiting added sugar intake is a much more practical and comprehensive approach. Later in this book, we'll explore a variety of healthy tips to improve your diet. And in the next few chapters, we are going to focus on some fundamental principles and rules about macronutrients – water, proteins, carbohydrates, and fats.

Water

You need water to live; over 50% of your body mass is made up of water. That means that water is the most important substance in our bodies. Among others, vital functions water facilitates digestion, removes waste and toxins, and regulates body temperature. Also, drinking enough water allows the liver to break down fat more efficiently.

37% of Americans often mistake thirst for hunger. This data means that they are eating instead of drinking when they are thirsty. Too much high-in-fat and high-in-sugar foods in menu provoke weakness of thirst sensitivity.

75% of Americans are dehydrated chronically; so it is a good idea to drink water regularly throughout the day. Start a new day with drinking water as soon as you wake, and end just before sleep. In the morning water increases your metabolism and in the evening drinking water decreases your hunger pangs.

There is no substitute for water, so you should drink water all the time. As a fitness enthusiast, you will need to drink even more water to replace fluids lost through transudation. Also, you need additional water to compensate for heat, alcohol, and caffeinated beverages.

So, how much water should you drink daily? Well, it depends; there is a valid test though. Keep an eye on the color of your urine and continue consuming water until your urine is clear or light yellow.

Protein

Protein is involved in building and repairing your cells and tissues. Also, adequate protein intake is essential for optimizing hormones and burning body fat. Protein typically consists of many amino acids; one of those amino acids – Phenylalanine triggers hormones that reduce hunger and stimulates weight loss. Even a single dose of Phenylalanine could decrease regular food intake, increase a level of appetite suppression hormone GLP-1, and diminish the level of the appetite-stimulating Ghrelin.

In general, your body doesn't want to change; it likes everything to stay the same. When you try to lose weight, your body will respond with compensation mechanisms like revving up your appetite-stimulating hormones.

That's why Atkins diet, Paleolithic diet, and others protein-rich diet plans could be useful in providing weight loss effect by making you feel full for longer period. Just adding more proteins to your menu can help you to reduce weight even without a complete nutritional revision. Our bodies cannot store protein, so you need some of it every day.

Proteins can be found in animals or plants. Yep, plants like soy, nuts, and seeds are rich in protein. Optimal protein intake is based on two factors: natural state and balanced intake.

Natural state means hormone-free, free-range, and organic products which have a better nutritional ratio and fewer detrimental factors. These sources are preferred forms of protein over powder and snack bar.

Balanced protein diet means a mix of lean meat, eggs, seafood, nuts, and seeds. By industry definition, meat can be considered lean if it has less than ten gram of total fat, less than four and a half gram of saturated fat, and less than ninety-five milligrams of cholesterol per 3.5-ounce serving. You can prepare lean meat or simply cut off all white visible fat before cooking. It's hard and not very efficient to trim excess fat from processed meats.

Most seafood is considered lean too. Actually, some fatty fish are not lean, but they are rich in heart-healthy Omega 3 fatty acids.

Both white and red meat has fat. The way you prepare the meat makes it lean. Even chicken can be high in fat, so remember to take the skin off because the skin adds a lot of fat. Also, broiling, grilling, roasting and baking are perfect cooking techniques which help cut down the fat content of meat.

Lean meat tends to be dry so marinate it with a small amount of oil, lemon juice and natural seasonings like herbs and spices. This trick makes lean meat more tender and juicy.

Carbohydrates

Carbohydrates provide human's body with its most favored form of energy but ingesting too many carbs will gain up body fat.

Vegetables, fruits, grain, cereal, pasta, anything with sugar, sugar itself are all carbohydrates. Naturally, we should moderate carbohydrates intake and focus on eating complex carbs and avoiding simple carbs. The main difference between complex and simple carbohydrates is how they impact on blood sugar level.

Simple carbohydrates break down too quickly and flood your blood with excessive sugar. In order to regulate the blood sugar, your body releases high amounts of hormone insulin into the blood. Insulin stops burning body's fat and instead, activates accumulating the unused sugar as fat. Growth hormone and insulin are competitors; that's why your evening meal shouldn't include simple carbs. Most of the growth hormone secretion occurs during sleep, and if insulin levels are high, GH can't access your cells.

One more hormone, adrenaline, which is released during intense physical activity, suppresses insulin. In this way, adrenaline creates a one-hour window when simple carbs can be consumed without increasing insulin. So if you consume simple carbohydrates at all, best do it after exercise.

The more simple carbs you eat, the more you crave them. Foods which contain simple carbohydrates are usually sweets, processed foods, starchy vegetables, and tropical fruits.

Complex carbohydrates provide a more constant flow of glucose into the bloodstream; that keeps you energized for longer. Also, eating complex carbs reduces hunger, helps you to eat less, declines risk of diabetes, and improves a level of blood cholesterol.

Fiber also is a type of carbohydrates; it's a substance in plants. However, we can't digest the fiber, so it passes through the entire intestine, mechanically cleaning it.

High-fiber food is good for human health, but most Americans don't eat enough fiber. Many studies show that fiber is a highly effective nutrient for losing weight. It slows down the movement and absorption of food. In this way, fiber keeps you satiated longer, maintains your blood sugar, and speeds up the process of eliminating toxins from your system. As we already know, the reason why many different fruits and vegetables have zero Smart-point is their high in fiber and relatively low-calorie count, which is perfect for weight loss.

Next to the veggies best sources of fiber include nuts, seeds, whole grains, cereals, and legumes. You may also read on a food label about soluble and insoluble fiber; both types are essential for health.

Soluble fiber lowers cholesterol levels, slows down the absorption of glucose, stabilizes insulin levels, and as a result causes you to eat less.

Insoluble fiber absorbs water, swells in the colon and removes toxic waste from there. One more function is to balance acidity in the intestines.

So, fiber helps eat less by acting as filler; it is also known to reduce the risk of diabetes, obesity, and heart attack. However, you should add fiber to your menu slowly over a period of a few weeks. This way allows bacterial flora in your digestive tract to adjust to the change. Increasing fiber consumption too quickly can lead to intestinal gas, abdominal bloating, and cramps.

And again, drink a plenty of water because fiber works better when it absorbs water.

As you see we shouldn't stop consuming carbohydrates; just choose the correct option. Get more of your carbohydrates from fruits and veggies; eat them raw with the skins for extra fiber. Eat whole fruit instead of drinking fruit juice. Eat more grains, nuts, and seeds.

Fats

Healthy fats are found in natural products like olives, avocados, seeds, nuts, fish, and animal proteins. Unhealthy fats are usually found in processed foods. Healthy fats provide energy, contribute to building cells and hormone optimization, and facilitate vitamin absorption. Probably, you have already consumed enough fats with your proteins. However, in order to lose weight, you should make differentiate between healthy and unhealthy fats.

Saturated fats are found in animal fat, like a full-fat dairy and fat on meat products. This type of fat is natural but you should limit your consumption. The reason for doing this is the fact that saturated fats increase the amount of harmful cholesterol in the blood and that leads to restricted blood flow. Another negative consequence is decreasing the body's efficiency in removing toxins from your blood.

Hydrogenated fats or trans-fats are the worst types of fats; you should avoid them as much as you can. Trans-fats consumption is strongly correlated with many health issues in general and heart problems in particular. This type of fat is used in processed foods to make them last longer. Also, it is found in packaged foods; store bought baked foods and fried foods.

Mono-unsaturated and polyunsaturated fats are best types of fats you can find. So, monounsaturated fat helps lower your LDL ("bad") cholesterol but still can lead to weight gain if consumed too much. Usually found in olive oil, peanut oil, and avocado oil.

Poly-unsaturated fats include two classes of fatty acids:

Omega-3 fatty acids are very healthy because they enhance the immune system and protect your cells and tissues against degenerative changes. We need omega-3 in our diet throughout the whole life for normal growth and development. In particular, Omega-3 affects the nervous system, brain development, IQ, and cognitive function. Great sources of Omega-3 fatty acids are pumpkin seeds, walnuts, flaxseed, fish and fish oil.

Omega-6 fatty acids are necessary for normal growth and development but still could be unhealthy in excessive quantities. It is also often over-consumed in the typical American diet, so you should keep a balance of your consumption. Usually found in sunflower, corn, sesame, and soy oils.

Mediterranean diet has a healthy balance of Omega-3 and Omega-6 fats which protects you from developing internal inflammation like obesity, cancer, Parkinson's, heart disease.

Also, you should know that many fat-free foods are high in sugar, so consuming them doesn't guarantee you are eating healthy. Avoiding fat could make provoke your overeating because fats help you feel full longer. The key is a proper balance between good fats and unhealthy fats. Also, you can limit saturated fats by trimming any fat you see around the meat before cooking.

FAT: Female Athlete Triad

For many active women and especially female athletes, the demands of eating low calorie/carbohydrate, a lot of training can combine with other normal life stressors such as relationships, jobs, and finances to shut the system down. However, a series of missed menstruation periods can be a really negative thing; don't take it lightly.

This issue happens so often that there is the syndrome named as "Female Athlete Triad" (FAT). Core symptoms of the syndrome include low energy, being without a period for three months, and decreased bone strength.

Apparently, woman's body is susceptible to deficiencies of energy, body fat or essential nutrients. Individual demands will vary from woman to woman. Some woman can eat fewer calories and work out with higher intensity and volume while staying hormonally healthy. For another woman, eating a restricted diet and/or strenuous exercising creates an unhappy hypothalamus, which is partly responsible for the hormones responsible for menstruation cycle. Hypothalamic amenorrhea is the scientific term for this.

Unless a woman plans to get pregnant, losing her period might seem like no big deal. You should remember that menstruation is not just about starting a family. In fact, it is a side effect of proper hormonal health. On the other side, having significant irregular periods means that something is wrong hormonally. In the case of above-mentioned hypothalamic amenorrhea, the production of hormones like progesterone and estrogen is dangerously reduced. It is a serious problem because your body needs these hormones for bone health. In fact, many health-conscious women who lose their menstruation end up with weak bones because of the link between progesterone, estrogen, and bone mineral density. Not rare that the first issue that drives women to the doctor is not the loss of period, but a terrible pain in one of their thighs, caused by a stress fracture.

Along with other hormones, estrogen and progesterone have wide-ranging effects throughout your body. That's why it's important to see your doctor; you could be dealing with some serious underlying issues. Also, in case that your cycle becomes irregular or stops altogether, you should increase calorie and carbohydrate intake by a little bit. Get enough rest and consider taking a high-quality multivitamin and mineral supplement. Mindset matters too, any type of stress makes things worse now. So, let your head relax.

Weight Loss Tips: More Small Changes

Eat before you get too hungry. And train yourself to stop before you get full. Slowly eating will make you enjoy the food more and feel fuller faster. It can take a while for our brain to confirm that we have had enough to eat. There are studies showing that chewing more slowly can increase the production of hormones associated with weight loss and help you eat fewer calories.

Don't binge late at night; calories are best ingested earlier in the day when you have more chances to work them off. Foods with the highest calorie content: junk food, processed food, salad dressings, and fried foods.

At each meal try to pick the healthful trio – including foods that deliver some protein, fat, and fiber. The protein will help you stay full for longer, the fat will work through the hormones to tell you to stop eating, and the fiber will make you feel full right away. Nuts and seeds are all smart choices as they have all three components.

For a strict weight loss diet, substitute grains with higher GI ratings such as rice, bread, and oatmeal for more veggies.

You should eat before you go shopping for food. You have to shop healthy because eating healthy is easier when you have not any junk food available. Write a grocery list before heading to the store; organize it by category in order to decrease your chances to purchase tempting unhealthy treats.

When you buy veggies and fruits, choose fresh or frozen options. Canned fruits and vegetables are nowhere near as nutritious and full of sugar and preservatives.

Often bad diet decisions are made when you have nothing healthy to eat in your kitchen. The easiest way to avoid unhealthy fats added sugar, and refined starches is to eat home-cooked foods. Find recipes you enjoy. If you don't like your meals, you will quit your diet plan and eat unhealthily.

Train planning and preparing healthy food in advance. This will save your time and make healthy eating easy and convenient. You won't have to make a choice when you are hungry and rushed.

Instead of removing certain food from your menu, try to substitute it with better and healthier alternatives. Think about what you can add to your diet plan, not what you have to avoid. This mindset helps you shift to a healthier way of life instead of restricting yourself from a particular food.

Focus on improving one meal each day. For instance, you might think about adding more nutrient-dense, whole foods. You can add protein, veggies, and fruits. Obviously, planning to eat less processed food and to drink fewer sweet drinks is a good move too. Once you have changed one meal a day, try another.

Sometimes your choices are limited. For example, when you are eating at a workplace cafeteria, or traveling. As a first-course order soup, then choose a salad and have lean protein for your main dish. Grilled chicken, turkey, or fish are smart choices. That way you will already be feeling full by the time your entrée arrives, making you less likely to overeat dessert.

Dining out and boozing can kill all your weight loss progress. Order your cocktail or glass of wine near the end of your meal; it will serve as a low-calorie dessert that way.

Caffeine can decrease water retention and increase energy. However, consuming too much caffeine regular makes you too used to it, and so the more you need for the same effect.

In fact, caffeine is a legal drug; please consume it moderately. Green tea contains caffeine and powerful antioxidants called catechins, which work synergistically with the caffeine to enhance fat burning.

For obvious reasons, portion control can be beneficial. Use the handful method to estimate your meal portion sizes. It's easy: one handful of protein plus one handful of carbohydrates plus two handfuls of leafy greens. One 4-oz. chicken breast is about the size of your hand, so it approximately equates to one handful of protein. Surely, the smaller person will have smaller palm and a smaller handful.

Just care more about what you are eating. Some studies show that keeping a food diary can help you lose more weight. You can simply take pictures of all your meals and later write down what you eat. Anything that increases your awareness of your food is likely to be helpful.

You shouldn't underrate the value of your night sleep. Studies show that sleep may be just as important as exercising and eating healthy. According to researchers, poor sleep is one of the most relevant risk factors for obesity. On the other hand, getting enough sleep can decrease your appetite by 14% and drop cravings for harmful food a 60%!

As we know, sugar is not proper food for weight loss. However, sugar-sweetened beverages are even worse. Sugar in liquid form is linked to a high risk of obesity. In fact, liquid calories may be the single most fattening aspect of your diet. You should remember that this applies to fruit juice too because juice contains a similar amount of sugar as a standard soft drink like coca-cola. Consume fruit juice with caution or simply avoid it altogether. Eat whole fruit instead.

Probably you already have heard that using smaller plates helps people automatically eat fewer calories. It seems to work, but here is an advanced option of this weird trick. Place veggies front and center on your plate, accompanied by sides of whole grains and protein. Usually, we think of meat or fish as our meal's main event; simply rearranging your plate helps automatically consume fewer calories and take in more vitamins and fiber.

Conclusion

Thank you again for downloading and reading this book! I hope you have gotten some new inspiration.

There is just so much to explore when it comes to the question of healthy nutrition. Many people are tired of looking for a diet which can help them to lose weight without making them feel exhausted. Try to focus on the making small changes in your lifestyle instead.

This book is just a guide. The next step is to actually implement some of these slight changes that you have learned. As you explore your own way of healthy eating, you will learn more tricks and tips, and start to understand how exactly it works in your unique case.

While diet seems to be the key factor to losing excess pounds, physical activity is critical for keeping the unwanted weight off. The workout can cause you to regain vitality and energy while losing weight. Dieters who regularly exercise report less stress, better sleep patterns, and fewer colds than those who don't exercise.